THE LYMPHATIC DIET COOKBOOK

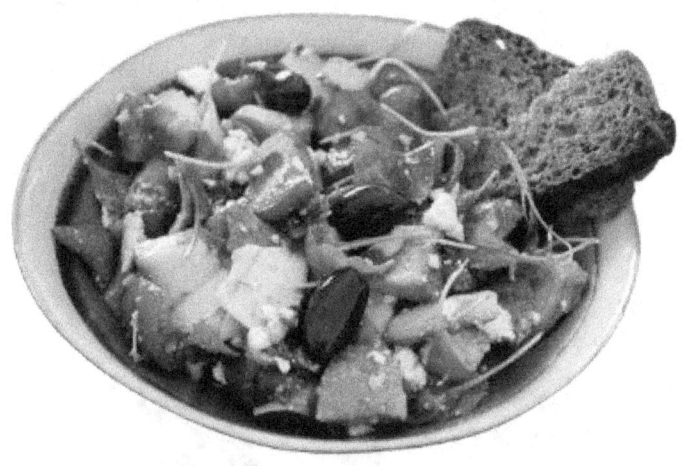

DR. Jessica Smith

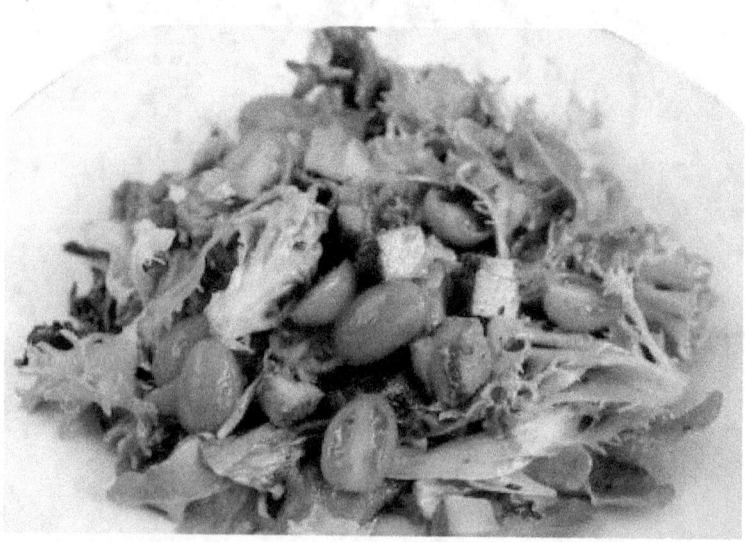

TABLE OF CONTENT

4

CHAPTER ONE

Introduction to the Lymphatic System

The lymphatic system, often referred to as the body's secondary circulatory system, plays a crucial role in maintaining overall health and well-being.

This intricate network of vessels, nodes, and organs functions as a key component of the immune system, contributing to the body's defense against infections, toxins, and other harmful substances.

At its core, the lymphatic system is responsible for the circulation and filtration of lymph, a colorless fluid containing white blood cells, proteins, and cellular waste products.

Unlike the circulatory system, which is closed and relies on the pumping action of the heart, the lymphatic system lacks a central pump. Instead, it depends on muscle contractions, breathing, and external movements to propel lymph through its vessels.

The lymphatic system acts as a drainage system, collecting excess fluid, known as lymphatic fluid or lymph, from the body's tissues and returning it to the bloodstream.

This process helps maintain fluid balance, preventing the accumulation of excess fluid in the tissues and reducing swelling. Beyond its role in fluid balance, the lymphatic system is a vital component of the body's immune defense mechanism.

Lymph nodes, small bean-shaped structures scattered throughout the system, act as filtering stations where foreign particles, pathogens, and damaged cells are captured and neutralized by specialized white blood cells.

Understanding the lymphatic system is fundamental to comprehending its impact on overall health. A well-functioning lymphatic system contributes to a robust immune response, efficient waste removal, and the prevention of chronic conditions associated with inflammation.

As we delve into the intricacies of the lymphatic system in this guide, we will explore how lifestyle, nutrition, and mindful practices can positively influence its function, promoting a state of holistic well-being.

The Role of the Lymphatic System in Health

The lymphatic system, often described as the unsung hero of the body, plays a multifaceted and indispensable role in maintaining optimal health.

While it may not receive as much attention as the cardiovascular system, its functions are paramount for the body's overall well-being.

Fluid Balance: One of the primary functions of the lymphatic system is to regulate fluid balance. It acts as a drainage system, collecting excess fluid from the interstitial spaces in tissues and returning it to the bloodstream.

This prevents the accumulation of fluids, reducing the risk of edema or swelling. Without this crucial function, tissues would become saturated, hindering cellular function and leading to discomfort and potential health complications.

Immune Defense: Perhaps the most vital role of the lymphatic system lies in its contribution to the body's immune defense. Lymph nodes, strategically positioned throughout the system, serve as hubs where immune cells, such as lymphocytes and macrophages, monitor and combat foreign invaders.

When harmful substances or pathogens enter the body, the lymphatic system responds by filtering and trapping these invaders in lymph nodes, initiating an immune response to neutralize and eliminate them. This defense mechanism is crucial for protecting the body against infections and illnesses.

Waste Removal: In addition to fluid and immune regulation, the lymphatic system is responsible for waste removal. Cellular waste, toxins, and byproducts are transported away from tissues and organs by lymphatic vessels.

This process ensures that metabolic waste is efficiently eliminated, preventing the buildup of harmful substances that could compromise cellular function and contribute to the development of diseases.

Fat Absorption: The lymphatic system is also involved in the absorption of dietary fats. Specialized vessels called lacteals in the small intestine absorb fats and fat-soluble vitamins, transporting them through the lymphatic system before entering the bloodstream. This function is crucial for nutrient absorption and overall metabolic health.

The lymphatic system is an integral component of the body's intricate network of systems. Its roles in fluid balance, immune defense, waste removal, and nutrient absorption collectively contribute to the maintenance of health and the prevention of various diseases.

A comprehensive understanding of the lymphatic system underscores its significance in promoting overall well-being and underscores the importance of adopting practices that support its optimal function.

Common Issues and Conditions Related to Lymphatic Health

The lymphatic system, a vital component of the immune and circulatory systems, is susceptible to various issues that can impact overall health. Understanding these common issues is essential for adopting preventive measures and promoting optimal lymphatic function.

Lymphedema: One of the primary concerns related to lymphatic health is lymphedema, a condition characterized by the swelling of tissues due to the accumulation of lymphatic fluid. This often occurs when lymph nodes are removed or damaged during cancer treatment, impeding the normal flow of lymph. Additionally, infections, trauma, or genetic factors can contribute to the development of lymphedema. Effective management involves specialized therapies, compression garments, and lifestyle modifications to alleviate symptoms and improve the quality of life for those affected.

Infections: Infections impacting the lymphatic system can lead to conditions like lymphangitis and lymphadenitis. Lymphangitis occurs when the lymphatic vessels become infected, causing red streaks and inflammation.

Lymphadenitis is an infection of the lymph nodes, resulting in swelling, tenderness, and sometimes the formation of pus-filled abscesses. Bacterial, viral, or fungal infections can trigger these conditions, and prompt medical attention is essential for proper diagnosis and treatment, often involving antibiotics.

Lymphomas: Lymphomas are cancers that originate in the lymphatic system, affecting lymphocytes, a type of white blood cell. Hodgkin lymphoma and non-Hodgkin lymphoma are the two main categories. These cancers can lead to swollen lymph nodes, fatigue, and other systemic symptoms.

Treatment may involve chemotherapy, radiation, and immunotherapy, depending on the specific type and stage of the lymphoma.

Autoimmune Disorders: Certain autoimmune disorders, such as rheumatoid arthritis and lupus, can impact the lymphatic system.

In these conditions, the immune system mistakenly attacks healthy tissues, including those within the lymphatic system, leading to inflammation and dysfunction. Managing the underlying autoimmune condition is crucial to mitigate the impact on lymphatic health.

Chronic Inflammation: Chronic inflammation is a common contributor to lymphatic issues. Inflammation can impair the normal flow of lymph, leading to fluid retention and compromised immune function.

Lifestyle factors, including poor diet, sedentary behavior, and stress, can contribute to chronic inflammation. Adopting an anti-inflammatory lifestyle, including a balanced diet and regular exercise, can help support lymphatic health.

Awareness of these common issues related to lymphatic health underscores the importance of proactive measures to maintain a well-functioning system.

Regular exercise, a balanced and nutritious diet, proper hydration, and prompt attention to any signs of infection or swelling are key components of a strategy to support optimal lymphatic function and overall well-being.

Overview of the Lymphatic Diet

The lymphatic diet is a nutritional approach designed to support the health and function of the lymphatic system, the body's network of vessels, nodes, and organs responsible for fluid balance and immune defense.

This diet emphasizes foods and lifestyle choices that promote optimal lymphatic function while minimizing factors that may contribute to inflammation and lymphatic congestion.

Hydration: Central to the lymphatic diet is adequate hydration. Proper water intake is crucial for maintaining the flow of lymphatic fluid, preventing dehydration-related issues, and supporting the body's detoxification processes.

14

Water helps flush out toxins and waste products, reducing the risk of lymphatic congestion.

Whole Foods and Antioxidants: The lymphatic diet emphasizes the consumption of whole, nutrient-dense foods rich in antioxidants.

Fruits and vegetables, particularly those with vibrant colors, provide essential vitamins, minerals, and antioxidants that support immune function and combat oxidative stress. Berries, leafy greens, citrus fruits, and cruciferous vegetables are particularly beneficial.

Healthy Fats: Incorporating healthy fats into the diet is another key aspect of lymphatic support. Omega-3 fatty acids, found in fatty fish, flaxseeds, and walnuts, have anti-inflammatory properties that can help reduce inflammation in the lymphatic system. Avocado, olive oil, and coconut oil are also valuable sources of healthy fats.

Herbs and Spices: Certain herbs and spices are known for their potential lymphatic benefits. Turmeric, ginger, and garlic, for example, have anti-inflammatory and immune-boosting properties. Including these spices in cooking can add flavor while providing potential health benefits.

Reducing Inflammatory Foods: The lymphatic diet advises minimizing or avoiding foods that may contribute to inflammation and lymphatic congestion.

This includes processed foods, refined sugars, excessive salt, and saturated fats. These substances can contribute to inflammation and may hinder the proper functioning of the lymphatic system.

Exercise and Movement: Beyond dietary considerations, the lymphatic diet emphasizes regular physical activity and movement.

Exercise promotes lymphatic circulation, helping to prevent stagnation and fluid buildup. Activities like walking, rebounding, and yoga can be particularly beneficial.

Stress Management: Stress can impact the immune system and overall health, including lymphatic function. The lymphatic diet encourages stress management techniques such as meditation, deep breathing exercises, and mindfulness practices to promote relaxation and reduce the negative effects of stress on the body.

The lymphatic diet is a holistic approach to supporting the lymphatic system through nutrition and lifestyle choices. By incorporating hydrating foods, antioxidants, healthy fats, and mindful practices, individuals can contribute to the overall health and function of their lymphatic system, fostering a state of well-being. It's essential to consult with healthcare professionals or nutritionists to tailor the diet to individual needs and conditions.

Foods That Support Lymphatic Function

The lymphatic system, integral to immune health and fluid balance, thrives when nourished with a diet rich in foods that promote optimal function. Incorporating certain nutrient-dense and anti-inflammatory foods can support lymphatic circulation, reduce inflammation, and enhance overall well-being.

1. Fruits and Vegetables: Colorful fruits and vegetables are nutritional powerhouses that provide essential vitamins, minerals, and antioxidants.

Berries, such as blueberries and strawberries, are particularly rich in antioxidants that combat oxidative stress and support immune function. Leafy greens, like spinach and kale, offer a plethora of nutrients, including vitamin C, which is crucial for immune health.

2. Citrus Fruits: Citrus fruits, such as oranges, lemons, and grapefruits, are excellent sources of vitamin C. Vitamin C plays a pivotal role in supporting the immune system and has antioxidant properties that may help reduce inflammation in the lymphatic system.

3. Omega-3 Fatty Acids: Fatty fish, flaxseeds, chia seeds, and walnuts are rich in omega-3 fatty acids. These essential fats have anti-inflammatory properties that can help reduce inflammation and support the overall health of the lymphatic system.

4. Herbs and Spices: Certain herbs and spices possess anti-inflammatory and immune-boosting properties. Turmeric, with its active compound curcumin, has been studied for its potential to reduce inflammation. Ginger and garlic are also known for their anti-inflammatory and immune-supportive effects.

5. Probiotic-Rich Foods: Probiotics, found in fermented foods like yogurt, kefir, sauerkraut, and kimchi, promote a healthy balance of gut bacteria.

A well-balanced gut microbiome is linked to a robust immune system, and supporting gut health indirectly contributes to lymphatic function.

6. Hydrating Foods: Maintaining proper hydration is essential for lymphatic function. Water-rich foods, such as watermelon, cucumber, and celery, contribute to overall hydration and assist in the movement of lymphatic fluid.

7. Herbal Teas: Certain herbal teas, like dandelion tea and green tea, are believed to have detoxifying properties that may support lymphatic function. Green tea, in particular, contains antioxidants known as catechins, which may have anti-inflammatory effects.

Incorporating these lymphatic-friendly foods into a well-balanced diet can contribute to the overall health of the lymphatic system.

It's important to note that individual dietary needs may vary, and consulting with healthcare professionals or nutritionists can provide personalized guidance for optimizing lymphatic function based on specific health conditions and preferences.

Foods to Avoid for a Healthy Lymphatic System

Maintaining a healthy lymphatic system involves not only choosing the right foods but also being mindful of those that may contribute to inflammation and hinder optimal function.

Certain dietary choices can impact the efficiency of the lymphatic system, potentially leading to congestion and compromised immune response. Here are some foods to consider minimizing or avoiding to support a healthy lymphatic system:

1. Processed Foods: Highly processed foods often contain artificial additives, preservatives, and excessive amounts of salt, which can contribute to inflammation. These foods lack the essential nutrients found in whole, unprocessed alternatives and may burden the lymphatic system with toxins and excess sodium.

2. Refined Sugars: Excessive consumption of refined sugars, commonly found in sweets, sugary beverages, and processed snacks, can lead to inflammation and may contribute to lymphatic congestion. High sugar intake has been linked to various health issues, including impaired immune function.

3. Saturated and Trans Fats: Foods high in saturated and trans fats, such as fried foods, processed snacks, and certain types of red meat, can contribute to inflammation and negatively impact cardiovascular health. These fats may impede the proper circulation of lymphatic fluid.

4. Excessive Salt: Consuming excessive amounts of salt can lead to water retention and swelling, potentially affecting lymphatic flow.

Processed and fast foods are often high in salt, so opting for fresh, whole foods and reducing added salt in cooking can help maintain a healthier balance.

5. Dairy Products: Some individuals may find that dairy products contribute to inflammation and mucus production, potentially impacting the lymphatic system. Experimenting with alternatives like almond or coconut milk may be beneficial for those sensitive to dairy.

6. Alcohol: Excessive alcohol consumption can compromise the liver, an organ crucial for detoxification and lymphatic function. Alcohol also dehydrates the body, potentially hindering the fluid balance necessary for optimal lymphatic operation.

7. Caffeine: While moderate caffeine intake is generally considered safe for many individuals, excessive caffeine consumption can lead to dehydration. Proper hydration is vital for lymphatic flow, so balancing caffeine intake with water consumption is recommended.

It's important to note that individual responses to these foods may vary, and dietary considerations should align with personal health conditions and preferences.

Adopting a balanced and varied diet, rich in whole foods and mindful of potential inflammatory triggers, can contribute to a healthier lymphatic system and overall well-being. Consulting with healthcare professionals or nutritionists can provide personalized guidance based on individual needs.

Mindful Eating and Its Impact on Lymphatic Health

Mindful eating, a practice rooted in awareness and attention to the present moment during meals, goes beyond simply choosing nutritious foods.

It encompasses the entire eating experience, from the selection and preparation of food to the act of consuming it.

This mindful approach has far-reaching implications for overall health, including potential benefits for the lymphatic system.

Connection to Digestive Health: Mindful eating encourages a heightened awareness of the eating process, including the taste, texture, and aroma of food. Chewing food thoroughly and savoring each bite aids in the breakdown of food particles in the mouth, initiating the digestive process.

Proper digestion is a crucial aspect of lymphatic health, as it ensures the efficient absorption of nutrients and the removal of waste products.

Reduced Stress Response: Chronic stress can negatively impact the lymphatic system by promoting inflammation and hindering immune function.

Mindful eating promotes a relaxed and focused state during meals, reducing the stress response associated with rushed or distracted eating. This, in turn, may contribute to a more balanced and resilient lymphatic system.

Support for Nutrient Absorption: Mindful eating encourages intentional and attentive consumption of nutrient-dense foods.

This practice supports the absorption of essential vitamins and minerals crucial for lymphatic health.

Nutrient-rich foods, when consumed with awareness, can provide the building blocks necessary for maintaining optimal lymphatic function.

Enhanced Hydration: Proper hydration is fundamental to lymphatic health, as it facilitates the movement of lymphatic fluid.

Mindful eating involves paying attention to thirst cues and choosing hydrating options, such as water-rich fruits and vegetables. Staying adequately hydrated supports the overall efficiency of the lymphatic system.

Prevention of Overeating: Mindful eating promotes a deeper connection with the body's hunger and fullness signals.

By tuning into these cues, individuals are less likely to overeat, preventing unnecessary strain on the digestive system and potentially reducing inflammation that could impact lymphatic function.

Emotional Well-Being: Emotional well-being is intricately connected to overall health, including lymphatic health. Mindful eating encourages a positive and non-judgmental approach to food, fostering a healthier relationship with eating. Emotional balance contributes to reduced stress, supporting a more resilient immune and lymphatic system.

CHAPTER TWO

Lymphatic Diet recipes

Breakfast

1. Berry Smoothie Bowl

Ingredients:

1 cup mixed berries (blueberries, strawberries, raspberries)

1 banana

1/2 cup low-fat yogurt

1 tablespoon chia seeds

1 tablespoon honey

Instructions:

Blend berries, banana, and yogurt until smooth.

Pour into a bowl and top with chia seeds and a drizzle of honey.

2. Avocado Toast with Smoked Salmon

Ingredients:

1 slice whole-grain bread

1/2 ripe avocado

50g smoked salmon

Lemon juice

Fresh dill

Instructions:

Toast the bread.

Mash the avocado and spread it on the toast.

Top with smoked salmon, a squeeze of lemon juice, and fresh dill.

3. Quinoa Breakfast Bowl

Ingredients:

1/2 cup cooked quinoa

1/4 cup Greek yogurt

1/2 cup mixed berries

1 tablespoon pumpkin seeds

Drizzle of maple syrup

Instructions:

Mix cooked quinoa with Greek yogurt.

Top with mixed berries, pumpkin seeds, and a drizzle of maple syrup.

4. Green Smoothie

Ingredients:

1 cup spinach

1/2 cucumber

1 green apple

1/2 lemon (juiced)

1 cup coconut water

Instructions:

Blend spinach, cucumber, green apple, lemon juice, and coconut water until smooth.

5. Oatmeal with Almond Butter and Banana

Ingredients:

1/2 cup rolled oats

1 cup almond milk

1 tablespoon almond butter

1 banana, sliced

Sprinkle of cinnamon

Instructions:

Cook rolled oats with almond milk.

Top with almond butter, banana slices, and a sprinkle of cinnamon.

6. Greek Yogurt Parfait

Ingredients:

1 cup Greek yogurt

1/2 cup granola

1/2 cup mixed berries

Drizzle of honey

Instructions:

Layer Greek yogurt with granola and mixed berries.

Drizzle with honey.

7. Chia Seed Pudding

Ingredients:

2 tablespoons chia seeds

1 cup almond milk

1/2 teaspoon vanilla extract

Sliced kiwi and strawberries

Instructions:

Mix chia seeds, almond milk, and vanilla extract. Let it sit in the fridge overnight.

Top with sliced kiwi and strawberries.

8. Coconut and Pineapple Smoothie

Ingredients:

1/2 cup coconut milk

1/2 cup pineapple chunks

1/2 banana

1 tablespoon shredded coconut

Instructions:

Blend coconut milk, pineapple, banana until smooth.

Top with shredded coconut.

9. Almond and Blueberry Pancakes

Ingredients:

1 cup almond flour

2 eggs

1/2 cup almond milk

1/2 cup blueberries

1/2 teaspoon baking powder

Instructions:

Mix almond flour, eggs, almond milk, and baking powder.

Cook pancakes, adding blueberries to each.

10. Spinach and Feta Omelet

Ingredients:

2 eggs

Handful of spinach

2 tablespoons feta cheese

Salt and pepper to taste

Instructions:

Whisk eggs and pour into a heated pan.

Add spinach and feta, fold, and cook until eggs are set.

11. Sweet Potato Hash with Poached Eggs
Ingredients:

1 sweet potato, grated

2 poached eggs

Fresh parsley

Salt and pepper to taste

Instructions:

Sauté grated sweet potato until tender.

Top with poached eggs, fresh parsley, salt, and pepper.

12. Brown Rice Porridge with Berries
Ingredients:

1/2 cup cooked brown rice

1/2 cup almond milk

1/4 cup mixed berries

1 tablespoon chopped nuts

Instructions:

Heat brown rice with almond milk.

Top with mixed berries and chopped nuts.

13. Tomato and Basil Breakfast Salad
Ingredients:

Cherry tomatoes, halved

Fresh basil leaves

1 tablespoon olive oil

Salt and pepper to taste

Poached eggs (optional)

Instructions:

Toss cherry tomatoes and basil with olive oil, salt, and pepper.

Top with poached eggs if desired.

14. Cottage Cheese and Pineapple Bowl

Ingredients:

1 cup cottage cheese

1/2 cup pineapple chunks

1 tablespoon sunflower seeds

Instructions:

Combine cottage cheese with pineapple chunks.

Sprinkle with sunflower seeds.

15. Buckwheat Pancakes with Mixed Berries

Ingredients:

1/2 cup buckwheat flour

1 egg

1/2 cup almond milk

Mixed berries for topping

Instructions:

Mix buckwheat flour, egg, and almond milk.

Cook pancakes and top with mixed berries.

Remember to tailor these recipes based on individual preferences and dietary needs. Additionally, consulting with a healthcare professional or nutritionist for personalized advice is recommended.

Lunch

1. Quinoa Salad with Avocado and Berries

Ingredients:

1 cup cooked quinoa

1 avocado, diced

1 cup mixed berries (blueberries, strawberries)

Handful of spinach leaves

1 tablespoon olive oil

Lemon juice, to taste

Salt and pepper, to taste

Instructions:

In a bowl, combine cooked quinoa, diced avocado, mixed berries, and spinach leaves.

Drizzle with olive oil and lemon juice. Toss gently to mix.

Season with salt and pepper to taste.

Serve chilled.

2. Grilled Salmon with Asparagus

Ingredients:

2 salmon fillets

1 bunch asparagus, trimmed

2 tablespoons olive oil

Lemon slices

Fresh dill, chopped

Salt and pepper, to taste

Instructions:

Preheat the grill. Season salmon with salt and pepper.

Brush asparagus with olive oil and season with salt.

Grill salmon and asparagus until cooked, turning occasionally.

Garnish with lemon slices and chopped dill before serving.

3. Lentil and Vegetable Soup

Ingredients:

1 cup lentils, rinsed

1 onion, diced

2 carrots, chopped

2 celery stalks, sliced

3 cloves garlic, minced

1 can diced tomatoes

6 cups vegetable broth

1 teaspoon cumin

Salt and pepper, to taste

Instructions:

In a large pot, sauté onion, carrots, celery, and garlic until softened.

Add lentils, diced tomatoes, vegetable broth, cumin, salt, and pepper.

Simmer until lentils are tender.

Adjust seasoning if needed and serve hot.

4. Spinach and Berry Salad with Grilled Chicken

Ingredients:

2 cups baby spinach

1 cup strawberries, sliced

1/2 cup blueberries

1 grilled chicken breast, sliced

1/4 cup feta cheese, crumbled

Balsamic vinaigrette dressing

Instructions:

Toss baby spinach, strawberries, blueberries, grilled chicken, and feta in a bowl.

Drizzle with balsamic vinaigrette dressing.

Gently toss until ingredients are well combined.

Serve immediately.

5. Cauliflower and Broccoli Stir-Fry

Ingredients:

2 cups cauliflower florets

2 cups broccoli florets

1 red bell pepper, sliced

1 cup snap peas

2 tablespoons soy sauce

1 tablespoon sesame oil

1 tablespoon rice vinegar

1 teaspoon ginger, minced

2 cloves garlic, minced

Instructions:

Heat sesame oil in a wok or skillet.

Stir-fry cauliflower, broccoli, bell pepper, and snap peas until crisp-tender.

In a small bowl, whisk together soy sauce, rice vinegar, ginger, and garlic.

Pour the sauce over the vegetables and toss until evenly coated.

Serve over brown rice or quinoa.

6. Turkey and Vegetable Lettuce Wraps

Ingredients:

1-pound ground turkey

1 onion, diced

1 bell pepper, diced

1 zucchini, grated

1 carrot, grated

Lettuce leaves for wrapping

2 tablespoons olive oil

1 teaspoon cumin

Salt and pepper, to taste

Instructions:

In a skillet, brown ground turkey in olive oil.

Add diced onion, bell pepper, grated zucchini, and carrot. Cook until vegetables are tender.

Season with cumin, salt, and pepper.

Spoon the mixture onto lettuce leaves, wrap, and enjoy.

7. Sweet Potato and Chickpea Buddha Bowl

Ingredients:

2 sweet potatoes, cubed

1 can chickpeas, drained and rinsed

2 cups kale, chopped

2 tablespoons olive oil

1 teaspoon paprika

1/2 teaspoon cumin

Salt and pepper, to taste

Tahini dressing

Instructions:

Toss sweet potatoes and chickpeas with olive oil, paprika, cumin, salt, and pepper.

Roast in the oven until golden and crispy.

Sauté kale in olive oil until wilted.

Assemble bowls with roasted sweet potatoes, chickpeas, and sautéed kale.

Drizzle with tahini dressing before serving.

8. Shrimp and Quinoa Stir-Fry

Ingredients:

1 cup quinoa, cooked

1-pound shrimp, peeled and deveined

1 bell pepper, sliced

1 cup broccoli florets

2 tablespoons soy sauce

1 tablespoon hoisin sauce

1 tablespoon sesame oil

1 teaspoon honey

1 tablespoon ginger, minced

Instructions:

In a wok or skillet, cook shrimp until pink and opaque. Set aside.

Stir-fry bell pepper and broccoli in sesame oil until crisp-tender.

In a small bowl, whisk together soy sauce, hoisin sauce, honey, and ginger.

Add cooked quinoa and shrimp to the vegetables. Pour the sauce over and toss until well combined.

Serve hot.

9. Mediterranean Chickpea Salad

Ingredients:

1 can chickpeas, drained and rinsed

1 cucumber, diced

1 cup cherry tomatoes, halved

1/2 red onion, finely chopped

1/4 cup Kalamata olives, sliced

Feta cheese, crumbled

Olive oil and balsamic vinegar

Fresh parsley, chopped

Salt and pepper, to taste

Instructions:

In a large bowl, combine chickpeas, cucumber, cherry tomatoes, red onion, and olives.

Drizzle with olive oil and balsamic vinegar.

Toss until well mixed. Season with salt and pepper.

Top with crumbled feta cheese and chopped parsley before serving.

10. Salmon and Vegetable Quinoa Bowl

Ingredients:

1 cup quinoa, cooked

2 salmon fillets

1 zucchini, sliced

1 yellow squash, sliced

1 cup cherry tomatoes, halved

2 tablespoons olive oil

Lemon slices

Fresh dill, chopped

Salt and pepper, to taste

Instructions:

Preheat the oven. Season salmon with salt and pepper.

Roast salmon, zucchini, yellow squash, and cherry tomatoes in olive oil until cooked.

Fluff cooked quinoa and divide into bowls.

Top with roasted salmon and vegetables. Garnish with lemon slices and chopped dill.

11. Vegetable and Tofu Stir-Fry

Ingredients:

1 block extra-firm tofu, cubed

2 cups broccoli florets

1 bell pepper, sliced

1 carrot, julienned

1 cup snap peas

2 tablespoons soy sauce

1 tablespoon hoisin sauce

1 tablespoon sesame oil

1 teaspoon ginger, minced

2 cloves garlic, minced

Instructions:

Press tofu to remove excess water, then cube it.

Sauté tofu in sesame oil until golden brown. Set aside.

Stir-fry broccoli, bell pepper, carrot, and snap peas until crisp-tender.

In a small bowl, whisk together soy sauce, hoisin sauce, ginger, and garlic.

Add tofu and sauce to the vegetables, tossing until well coated.

Serve over brown rice or quinoa.

12. Chicken and Vegetable Brown Rice Bowl

Ingredients:

1 cup brown rice, cooked

1 chicken breast, grilled and sliced

1 cup broccoli florets

1 bell pepper, diced

1 carrot, sliced

2 tablespoons soy sauce

1 tablespoon olive oil

1 teaspoon honey

1 teaspoon garlic, minced

Instructions:

In a pan, sauté broccoli, bell pepper, and carrot in olive oil until tender.

Add sliced grilled chicken to the vegetables.

In a small bowl, mix soy sauce, honey, and minced garlic. Pour over the chicken and vegetables.

Serve over cooked brown rice.

13. Zoodle Salad with Pesto Chicken

Ingredients:

2 zucchinis, spiralized into zoodles

1 cup cherry tomatoes, halved

1/4 cup pine nuts, toasted

1/2 cup grilled chicken, sliced

Fresh basil leaves

Pesto sauce

Lemon juice

Salt and pepper, to taste

Instructions:

In a bowl, combine zoodles, cherry tomatoes, pine nuts, and grilled chicken.

Drizzle with pesto sauce and lemon juice. Toss gently to mix.

Season with salt and pepper to taste.

Garnish with fresh basil leaves before serving.

14. Black Bean and Corn Salad

Ingredients:

1 can black beans, drained and rinsed

1 cup corn kernels (fresh or frozen)

1 red bell pepper, diced

1/2 red onion, finely chopped

Fresh cilantro, chopped

Lime juice

2 tablespoons olive oil

Cumin, to taste

Salt and pepper, to taste

Instructions:

In a large bowl, combine black beans, corn, bell pepper, and red onion.

Drizzle with olive oil and lime juice.

Add chopped cilantro and season with cumin, salt, and pepper.

Toss until well combined. Serve chilled.

15. Eggplant and Chickpea Curry

Ingredients:

1 eggplant, diced

1 can chickpeas, drained and rinsed

1 onion, diced

2 tomatoes, diced

2 cloves garlic, minced

1 tablespoon curry powder

1 teaspoon turmeric

1 teaspoon cumin

1 can coconut milk

Fresh cilantro, chopped

Salt and pepper, to taste

Instructions:

Sauté diced eggplant, onion, and garlic in a pan until softened.

Add chickpeas, tomatoes, curry powder, turmeric, and cumin. Stir well.

Pour in coconut milk and simmer until the sauce thickens.

Season with salt and pepper. Garnish with chopped cilantro before serving.

Serve over quinoa or brown rice.

Dinner

1. Lemon Herb Grilled Salmon:

Ingredients:

4 salmon fillets

2 tablespoons olive oil

1 lemon (juiced)

2 cloves garlic (minced)

Fresh herbs (rosemary, thyme, and parsley), chopped

Salt and pepper to taste

Instructions:

In a bowl, mix olive oil, lemon juice, minced garlic, and chopped herbs.

Marinate salmon fillets in the mixture for 30 minutes.

Grill salmon until cooked through, approximately 4-5 minutes per side.

Season with salt and pepper before serving.

2. Quinoa and Vegetable Stir-Fry:

Ingredients:

1 cup quinoa

2 cups mixed vegetables (broccoli, bell peppers, carrots)

2 tablespoons low-sodium soy sauce

1 tablespoon sesame oil

2 cloves garlic (minced)

1 teaspoon fresh ginger (grated)

Instructions:

Cook quinoa according to package instructions.

In a wok, stir-fry mixed vegetables in sesame oil until tender.

Add minced garlic and grated ginger, then stir in cooked quinoa.

Drizzle with soy sauce and toss until well combined.

3. Roasted Chicken with Sweet Potatoes:
Ingredients:

4 boneless, skinless chicken breasts

2 sweet potatoes, peeled and diced

2 tablespoons olive oil

1 teaspoon dried thyme

1 teaspoon paprika

Salt and pepper to taste

Instructions:

Preheat oven to 400°F (200°C).

In a bowl, toss sweet potatoes with olive oil, thyme, and paprika.

Season chicken breasts with salt and pepper, place on a baking sheet, and surround with sweet potatoes.

Roast for 25-30 minutes or until chicken is cooked through.

4. Spinach and Chickpea Salad:

Ingredients:

4 cups fresh spinach

1 can (15 oz) chickpeas, drained and rinsed

1 cucumber, diced

1 cup cherry tomatoes, halved

2 tablespoons balsamic vinaigrette

Feta cheese (optional)

Instructions:

In a large bowl, combine spinach, chickpeas, cucumber, and cherry tomatoes.

Drizzle with balsamic vinaigrette and toss to coat.

Top with crumbled feta cheese if desired.

5. Turkey and Vegetable Skewers:

Ingredients:

1 lb turkey breast, cut into cubes

Bell peppers (red, yellow, and green), cut into chunks

Red onion, cut into wedges

Zucchini, sliced

Olive oil

Garlic powder, onion powder, paprika, salt, and pepper to taste

Instructions:

Preheat grill or oven.

Thread turkey, bell peppers, red onion, and zucchini onto skewers.

Brush with olive oil and sprinkle with seasonings.

Grill for 12-15 minutes, turning occasionally until turkey is cooked.

6. Lentil and Vegetable Soup:

Ingredients:

1 cup dried lentils

4 cups vegetable broth

2 carrots, diced

2 celery stalks, diced

1 onion, chopped

2 cloves garlic, minced

1 teaspoon cumin

1 teaspoon turmeric

Salt and pepper to taste

Instructions:

Rinse lentils and combine with vegetable broth in a pot.

Add carrots, celery, onion, garlic, cumin, turmeric, salt, and pepper.

Simmer for 25-30 minutes until lentils are tender.

7. Baked Cod with Herbed Quinoa:

Ingredients:

4 cod fillets

1 cup quinoa

2 cups chicken or vegetable broth

2 tablespoons chopped fresh dill

1 lemon (sliced)

Olive oil

Salt and pepper to taste

Instructions:

Preheat oven to 375°F (190°C).

Rinse quinoa and cook in broth according to package instructions.

Place cod fillets on a baking sheet, drizzle with olive oil, and season with salt and pepper.

Bake for 15-18 minutes, or until the cod is cooked through.

Serve over a bed of herbed quinoa, garnished with fresh dill and lemon slices.

8. Avocado and Chickpea Salad:

Ingredients:

2 avocados, diced

1 can (15 oz) chickpeas, drained and rinsed

Cherry tomatoes, halved

Red onion, finely chopped

Fresh cilantro, chopped

Lime juice

Salt and pepper to taste

Instructions:

In a bowl, combine diced avocados, chickpeas, cherry tomatoes, and red onion.

Drizzle with lime juice and sprinkle with cilantro, salt, and pepper.

Gently toss to combine.

9. Stir-Fried Tofu with Broccoli:

Ingredients:

1 block firm tofu, cubed

2 cups broccoli florets

2 tablespoons soy sauce

1 tablespoon sesame oil

1 tablespoon rice vinegar

2 cloves garlic, minced

1 teaspoon fresh ginger, grated

Green onions, chopped (for garnish)

Instructions:

Press tofu to remove excess water and cut into cubes.

In a wok or pan, stir-fry tofu until golden.

Add broccoli, garlic, and ginger, and stir-fry until broccoli is tender-crisp.

Drizzle with soy sauce, sesame oil, and rice vinegar, tossing to coat.

Garnish with chopped green onions before serving.

10. **Shrimp and Asparagus Stir-Fry:**

Ingredients:

1 lb shrimp, peeled and deveined

1 bunch asparagus, trimmed and cut into pieces

2 tablespoons low-sodium soy sauce

1 tablespoon hoisin sauce

1 tablespoon olive oil

2 cloves garlic, minced

1 teaspoon sesame seeds (optional)

Instructions:

In a wok or pan, sauté shrimp and asparagus in olive oil until shrimp is cooked.

Add minced garlic and continue to stir-fry for another minute.

Drizzle with soy sauce and hoisin sauce, tossing to coat.

Sprinkle with sesame seeds before serving.

11. Mediterranean Chickpea Salad:

Ingredients:

2 cans (15 oz each) chickpeas, drained and rinsed

Cucumber, diced

Cherry tomatoes, halved

Kalamata olives, sliced

Red onion, finely chopped

Feta cheese, crumbled

Olive oil

Lemon juice

Fresh oregano, chopped

Instructions:

In a large bowl, combine chickpeas, cucumber, cherry tomatoes, olives, and red onion.

Drizzle with olive oil and lemon juice, then toss to combine.

Top with crumbled feta cheese and chopped fresh oregano.

12. Broccoli and Chicken Stir-Fry:

Ingredients:

2 boneless, skinless chicken breasts, thinly sliced

2 cups broccoli florets

1 bell pepper, sliced

2 tablespoons soy sauce

1 tablespoon honey

1 tablespoon cornstarch

1 tablespoon sesame oil

2 cloves garlic, minced

Cooked brown rice (optional, for serving)

Instructions:

In a bowl, mix soy sauce, honey, and cornstarch to create a sauce.

In a wok or pan, stir-fry chicken until cooked through.

Add broccoli, bell pepper, and minced garlic, continuing to stir-fry until vegetables are tender-crisp.

Pour the sauce over the chicken and vegetables, tossing to coat.

Drizzle with sesame oil and serve over brown rice if desired.

13. Tomato Basil Zucchini Noodles:

Ingredients:

4 medium zucchinis, spiralized into noodles

2 cups cherry tomatoes, halved

1/4 cup fresh basil, chopped

2 tablespoons olive oil

2 cloves garlic, minced

Red pepper flakes (optional)

Parmesan cheese (optional, for garnish)

Instructions:

In a pan, sauté zucchini noodles in olive oil until tender.

Add cherry tomatoes, minced garlic, and red pepper flakes (if using).

Cook for an additional 2-3 minutes, then stir in fresh basil.

Garnish with Parmesan cheese before serving.

14. Baked Eggplant Parmesan:

Ingredients:

2 large eggplants, sliced

2 cups marinara sauce

1 cup mozzarella cheese, shredded

1/2 cup Parmesan cheese, grated

1 cup whole wheat breadcrumbs

2 tablespoons olive oil

Fresh basil, chopped (for garnish)

Instructions:

Preheat oven to 375°F (190°C).

Dip eggplant slices in olive oil, then coat with breadcrumbs.

Arrange the slices on a baking sheet and bake for 20 minutes.

In a baking dish, layer baked eggplant with marinara sauce and cheese.

Bake for an additional 20-25 minutes until cheese is melted and bubbly.

Garnish with fresh basil before serving.

15. Lentil and Spinach Stuffed Bell Peppers:

Ingredients:

4 bell peppers, halved and seeds removed

1 cup dried green lentils

2 cups vegetable broth

1 onion, diced

2 cloves garlic, minced

2 cups fresh spinach, chopped

1 can (15 oz) diced tomatoes

1 teaspoon cumin

1 teaspoon paprika

Salt and pepper to taste

Instructions:

Preheat oven to 375°F (190°C).

Rinse lentils and cook in vegetable broth until tender.

In a pan, sauté onion and garlic until softened.

Add chopped spinach, diced tomatoes, cumin, paprika, salt, and pepper, and cook until spinach is wilted.

Stir in cooked lentils.

Stuff halved bell peppers with the lentil and spinach mixture.

Bake for 25-30 minutes until peppers are tender.

Snack

1. Berry Bliss Smoothie Bowl

Ingredients:

1 cup mixed berries (strawberries, blueberries, raspberries)

1 banana

1/2 cup Greek yogurt

1 tablespoon chia seeds

1 tablespoon honey

Instructions:

Blend mixed berries, banana, and Greek yogurt until smooth.
Pour into a bowl, top with chia seeds, and drizzle with honey.

2. Avocado and Tomato Rice Cakes

Ingredients:

2 rice cakes

1 ripe avocado, mashed

1 tomato, sliced

Sprinkle of sea salt and black pepper

Fresh cilantro for garnish

Instructions:

Spread mashed avocado evenly on rice cakes. Top with
sliced tomatoes, season with salt and pepper, and garnish
with fresh cilantro.

3. Cucumber Hummus Boats

Ingredients:

2 large cucumbers

1 cup hummus

Cherry tomatoes, sliced

Fresh parsley, chopped

Instructions:

Cut cucumbers in half lengthwise. Scoop out seeds to create "boats." Fill each boat with hummus and top with sliced cherry tomatoes and chopped parsley.

4. Quinoa and Vegetable Stuffed Peppers
Ingredients:

3 bell peppers, halved

1 cup cooked quinoa

1/2 cup cherry tomatoes, halved

1/4 cup cucumber, diced

Fresh basil, chopped

Instructions:

Combine cooked quinoa, cherry tomatoes, cucumber, and fresh basil. Spoon the mixture into halved bell peppers.

5. Almond Butter Banana Bites

Ingredients:

2 bananas, sliced

Almond butter

Chia seeds

Instructions:

Spread almond butter on banana slices and sprinkle with chia seeds. Stack slices to create banana bites.

6. Greek Yogurt Parfait

Ingredients:

1 cup Greek yogurt

1/2 cup granola

Mixed berries (strawberries, blueberries)

Honey for drizzling

Instructions:

Layer Greek yogurt, granola, and mixed berries in a glass. Drizzle with honey.

7. Edamame and Sea Salt

Ingredients:

1 cup edamame, steamed

Sea salt to taste

Instructions:

Steam edamame and sprinkle with sea salt for a protein-packed, simple snack.

8. Zucchini Noodles with Pesto

Ingredients:

1 large zucchini, spiralized

2 tablespoons pesto

Cherry tomatoes, halved

Instructions:

Toss zucchini noodles with pesto and top with cherry tomatoes.

9. Apple Slices with Nut Butter

Ingredients:

1 apple, sliced

Almond or peanut butter

Instructions:

Spread nut butter on apple slices for a satisfying and crunchy snack.

10. Chia Seed Pudding
Ingredients:

3 tablespoons chia seeds

1 cup almond milk

Fresh berries for topping

Instructions:

Mix chia seeds and almond milk. Let it sit in the refrigerator for a few hours or overnight. Top with fresh berries before serving.

11. Carrot and Hummus Dippers
Ingredients:

2 large carrots, sliced

1/2 cup hummus

Instructions:

Dip carrot slices into hummus for a nutritious and crunchy snack.

12. Spinach and Feta Stuffed Mushrooms

Ingredients:

8 large mushrooms, cleaned and stems removed

1 cup spinach, chopped

1/4 cup feta cheese, crumbled

Instructions:

Mix chopped spinach and feta, then stuff the mushrooms. Bake until mushrooms are tender.

13. Mango Salsa with Jicama Chips

Ingredients:

1 ripe mango, diced

1/2 red onion, finely chopped

Fresh cilantro, chopped

Jicama, sliced into chips

Instructions:

Combine diced mango, chopped red onion, and cilantro. Serve with jicama chips.

14. Roasted Chickpeas

Ingredients:

1 can chickpeas, drained and rinsed

1 tablespoon olive oil

1 teaspoon paprika

Sea salt to taste

Instructions:

Toss chickpeas with olive oil, paprika, and sea salt. Roast in the oven until crispy.

15. Watermelon and Mint Skewers

Ingredients:

Watermelon, cut into cubes

Fresh mint leaves

Wooden skewers

Instructions:

Thread watermelon cubes and mint leaves onto skewers for a refreshing and hydrating snack.

CONCLUSION

In embracing the principles of the lymphatic diet, we embark on a journey toward holistic well-being, recognizing that the choices we make in our kitchens profoundly impact the intricate workings of our bodies.

This culinary exploration, designed with lymphatic health in mind, extends beyond mere sustenance. It becomes a deliberate and thoughtful approach to nourishing the body, supporting the immune system, and fostering a sense of vitality.

As we conclude this gastronomic voyage, let us carry forward the understanding that the lymphatic system, our silent guardian, thrives on a symphony of nutrient-rich foods, hydration, and mindful practices.

Each recipe within these pages represents a harmonious blend of flavors, textures, and nutrients carefully curated to not only tantalize the taste buds but also to fortify the body's natural defenses.

May these culinary creations inspire a shift in perspective, encouraging a connection with the nourishing essence of every ingredient.

Let the vibrant hues of fruits and vegetables, the richness of healthy fats, and the simplicity of hydration become not just components of a meal but integral elements of a lymphatic-friendly lifestyle.

Through this conscious approach to eating, we empower ourselves to promote lymphatic circulation, reduce inflammation, and enhance overall health.

As we savor these recipes, let us revel in the knowledge that we are partaking in a feast that extends beyond the plate—a feast for the lymphatic system, a celebration of wellness, and a commitment to nourishing our bodies with the care they truly deserve.

May these recipes serve as a catalyst for a sustained and mindful relationship with food, encouraging a lifelong dedication to the well-being of both body and spirit. Cheers to a lymphatic diet that not only delights the palate but also elevates our understanding of the profound connection between nutrition and vitality.